Is Becoming A Certified Nursing Assistant for Me?

Cedric Jackson

Disclaimer

The information contained in this book is meant to serve as a comprehensive collection of ideas and tips. Summaries, strategies, tips and tricks are only recommendations by the author, and reading this Book does not guarantee that one's results will exactly mirror our own results. The author of this book made all reasonable efforts to provide current and accurate information for the readers of this Book. The authors will not be held liable for any unintentional errors or omissions that may be found.

The material in this book may include information, products, or services by third parties. As such, the author of this guide does not assume responsibility or liability for any Third Party Material or opinions.

The publication of such Third Party materials does not constitute the authors' guarantee of any information, instruction, opinion, products or service contained within the Third Party Material. Use of recommended Third Party Material does not guarantee that your results will mirror our own. Publication of such Third Party Material is simply a recommendation and expression of the authors' own opinion of that material.

Dedication

I dedicate this book to all the certified nursing assistants around the world, who have devoted themselves to providing excellent day-to-day care to their clients and for their heartfelt kindness, relentless dedication and unswerving devotion to providing compassionate care and improving the quality of life all persons in their care.

Thank you!

~Cedric J.

Table of Contents

Preface

Why did I choose to enter the Healthcare field to become a certified nursing assistant? To best answer that question, I would like to share with you my own personal testimony and I hope that it will inspire and motivate you to consider entering the Healthcare field to become a certified nursing assistant.

My First Job as a Nursing Assistant—Volunteers of America—$7.00 an hour!

It was in the fall of 99' that I would attend Rhema Bible College—a seminary school located in the beautiful city of Broken Arrow, Oklahoma, where I would receive my ministerial training and education for ministry.

After settling in to ministry school and my new apartment in Broken Arrow, I had strict plans to find a job that would provide me with a nice income and ample time for my studies; therefore I prayed the night before that God would lead me to such a job.

The next morning I woke up early, said a short prayer, and purchased a newspaper and off I went to find a job.

I made numerous calls to various companies, but inwardly I felt none of those were the places that God would have me to apply to, so I kept praying and looking.

It was nearing evening time and I was getting very exhausted and weary with job hunting as I had been searching all morning, afternoon and into the evening. Then all of a sudden as I was driving down the highway, my eyes seemed to magically gaze upward and to the right side of the road, where a large sign read—"Volunteers of America – Now Hiring Nursing Assistants / $7.00 an hour, Apply Now!" Immediately, I felt in my heart, God say, "Apply here, this is where I want you to work!"

I exclaimed "Lord!", as my heart began to sink into my chest, "How am I going to pay for my schooling, rent, utility bills and groceries on $7.00 an hour?", "How, Lord?". I've never worked in the Healthcare field, yet all I felt on the inside was, "Trust Me!"

It would be nice to say that I obediently obeyed my Lord's will, but sadly I didn't. I drove off and tried my best to get far away as I could from that place. I made every turn I could. I turned to the right. I turned to the left. I went straight and just when I thought, I was thoroughly lost and away from that place, what appeared to my right as I drove down the road made me sigh. It was that same sign I had passed earlier, that still read the same—"Volunteers of America – Now Hiring Nursing Assistants \ $7.00 an hour, Apply Now". But now it seemed that the 'Apply Now!' was in bold print, highlighted and underlined. I chuckled a bit as I dropped my head and said, "Okay, okay Lord thine will be done". I sheepishly went into Volunteers of America and asked for an application and got hired on the spot.

I Was a Changed Man after my First Client

My first client at Volunteers of America, whom I will call Tim (*not real name for protection*), was a most memorable and unforgettable one, who totally gave me a new perspective and a new heart on what it meant to be a caregiver.

Although Tim suffered with many health problems such as Cerebral Palsy, seizures, speech impediments and foot deformities, he was the nicest and most respectful person you would ever want to meet.

We developed such a close friendship and I was proud to say I was his friend. A friendship that I'll never forget. We ate together, watched movies, cooked out, went to baseball games, parks, fairs, put together puzzles, and the list goes on and on. We also faced many challenges with his health issues but we made it through them.

If there was a downside from working at Volunteers of America with Tim, it was when our paths parted due to me moving back home, after completing my ministerial training at Rhema Bible College. Nevertheless, it was an experience that I'll never forget. It was there that I truly began to understand what it meant to be a servant.

Why I wrote this Book?

When I became a nursing assistant, there were many questions that I had and many things that I wished I knew, while in this field, but didn't. So this prompted to me to write this book and to help guide and inform you of the many things that I wish I had known. For example, how do you become certified, what steps to take, what are all the different type of jobs that are available for certified nursing assistants, etc.

So it's my intent to cover these and many other questions that you may have so that you can confidently pursue a career as a certified nursing assistant.

And since I have been in this field for many years and have learned many things from many people, I felt it only right to share with you my own personal knowledge, experience and research in my new and exciting Book—"Is Becoming a Certified Nursing Assistant for Me?"

Certified Nursing Assistant
&
BLS/HIV/Dementia/First Aid Certified

Cedric Jackson

Introduction

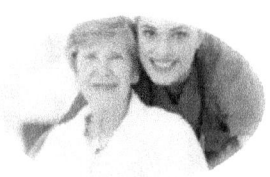

Congratulations on taking this crucial step in determining if becoming a certified nursing assistant is right for you, by purchasing my informative Book, entitled—"Is Becoming a Certified Nursing Assistant for Me?"

In this informative Book, I will help guide you in deciding if becoming a certified nursing assistant is right for you, by answering and discussing the following:

- What character traits are a must for certified nursing assistants?
- Why are these character traits important?
- What are these character traits?
- What are the steps in becoming a certified nursing assistant?
- How much will it cost to become a certified nursing assistant and how long will it take to complete a program?
- Are there other certifications required for employment?
- What are the different areas that a certified nursing assistant can work in?
- What is the job outlook for certified nursing assistants?
- What is the pay rate for certified nursing assistants?
- What are some tips for job interviews?
- How do you become a self-employed certified nursing assistant?
- What if you desire to advance to a LPN or RN?

Along with this Book, I've also developed a website at www.cnanationwide.com, which was developed with the intent to cater to three specific groups of people, and they are as follows:

1. Potential certified nursing assistants.
2. Nursing assistants in training to become certified nursing assistants.
3. Certified nursing assistants that would like to advance to LPNs or RNs.

I will be making reference to this website throughout this book, so please feel free to visit and become a member of cnanationwide.com, which is absolutely free, by using the sign-up form on the site. Also feel free to download our free resource guide, "Resource Guide: CNA Employment Opportunities".

It's my desire, that by the end of this book, you will have come to a definitive decision on whether or not you should pursue a career as a certified nursing assistant.

Now, let's get started, because I have lots of information to share with you!

Chapter 1. What Character Traits are a Must for Certified Nursing Assistants?

"Character is Destiny." - Heraclitus

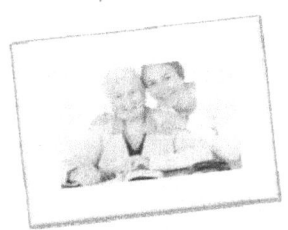 If you are considering a career as a certified nursing assistant, then one of the most important questions to ask yourself is, "Do I have the character traits of a certified nursing assistant?"

Now, you may be asking yourself, "What are these character traits and why are they important when considering a career as a certified nursing assistant?"

The possessing of these character traits, in which I will cover momentarily, are important for a number of reasons.

The first being, a majority of employers list these character traits as necessary qualifications for employment, because they thoroughly understand the nature of the job of being a certified nursing assistant, and what type of person it takes to be a successful one.

Furthermore, employers are very protective of their clients, whether they are elderly or disabled, and by selecting candidates who possess these set of traits, it thereby lowers the risk of hiring someone that could potentially bring harm instead of help to their clients.

Lastly, it allows for you to honestly and objectively assess your own personality and character traits, to determine if you would make a good certified nursing assistant or not.

So, this leaves us with the question, "What are these character traits?"

The Seven Character Traits That You Must Possess

Character Trait 1 - You Must Be Empathetic

If you are considering entering the Health Care field to become a certified nursing assistant then you must be empathetic. Where being *empathetic* simply means, *a person who can share in another person's feelings (particularly of the clients (the elderly and disabled))* or more simply put, putting yourself in the other person's shoes, to try and gain insight and understanding of their particular situations.

Possessing this trait of being empathetic is important, particularly in the Healthcare Field as a certified nursing assistant. When you practice empathy by placing yourself in your client's shoes and seeing things as they see them, it provides you with more objectivity—seeing things from their perspective without interjecting your own opinions or feelings. This allows you to accurately assess situations because your assessments are based on facts obtained from your client and not your own personal opinions. This accurate assessment, based on facts, leads to effective solutions by precisely knowing what problems needs to be solved and what issues needs to be addressed.

I really can't stress enough of how important being empathetic is in working with the elderly and disabled, because there will be many clients that you will not be able to thoroughly understand and help, until you are able to practice being empathetic towards them.

One classic example of empathy can clearly be seen through an experiment called,
"Experience 12 Minutes in Alzheimer's Dementia".

ABC Television's News Anchor, Cynthia McFadden followed a couple from Texas: Blaine Wilson, his wife and his mother—Lawanda that had Alzheimer's for four years. Cynthia's goal was to study the effects of Lawanda's

Alzheimer's on the family by filming on location and interviews.

During this four years an Alzheimer's simulation was constructed to allow the News anchor, Cynthia McFadden and Blain Wilson the son, to experience what is what like to have Alzheimer's. Prior to this experiment that weren't very empathetic towards Lawanda, but afterwards they were very empathetic because they experienced it for themselves, which left them with a greater understanding of the day-to-day challenges of an Alzheimer's victim. As a result of Blaine's new found empathy, he was able to provide better care with greater patience than before. To see this video, click on the following link:

<u>Experience 12 Minutes in Alzheimer's Dementia</u>.
(https://youtu.be/LL_Gq7Shc-Y)

Character Trait 2 - You Must Have Patience

In working with the elderly and the disabled, possessing the character trait of patience is an absolute must, where patience is defined as, *"the state of endurance under difficult circumstances, which can mean preserving in the face of delay or provocation without acting on negative annoyance/anger;"*. Being consistently aware of the fact that elderly and disabled clients may suffer from one or more disabilities or ailments is important in being patient, especially in providing day-to-day care. These disabilities or ailments such as: hearing and vision impairments, dementia, knee and back problems, and even debilitating arthritis can make even the most easiest of task, difficult to perform; therefore by being patient in providing care, the client is able to be put at ease by not being rushed or pushed, which could easily result in an unnecessary injury.

Character Trait 3 - You Must Possess Strong Communication Skills

The ability to communicate clearly and accurately to clients is an important trait to possess.

When communicating to the elderly, it is important to do three things in your communication and they are: be decisive, clear and to the point.

To be decisive is to know exactly what it is that you want to communicate. Knowing exactly what you want to communicate, comes from being perfectly clear in your own mind, what it is you want to say or what it is you would like for them to do. If you are not decisive it will appear that you really don't know what you are doing and this is the last thing that you want to convey, especially when they are depending on you. Your decisiveness will relay to them confidence in your abilities.

Secondly, you must be clear in what you want to say. What I mean by being is clear is not being too wordy in what you want to communicate. It's best to use words that are specific and refrain from using too many unnecessary words, which leads me to the last thing and that is being to the point. You don't want to beat around the bush, just be precise by getting directly to the point.

Character Trait 4 - You Must Be Observant

Being observant is vitally important in the overall safety of clients in their daily lives. It's vitally important because as we age our bodies undergoes degeneration to varying degrees. The rate of degeneration is not the same in all people, but for the most part the sight, touch, smell, taste and hearing will all be affected in some way. Therefore, due to degeneration, clients will depend on you for their sight, touch, taste, smell and feel, which is critically when it comes to their overall safety. You will have to engage your senses and be able to notice not only things that are right but things that are wrong.

It's easy to observe and take note of things that are right, but it takes stronger and more focused observant skills to intentionally look for things that are wrong. For instance is there water spillage on the floor which could cause slips, or are there missing parts on equipment (wheel chair, Hoyer lift, walker, etc.), or is the food in the refrigerator expired, etc.

Your keenness in being observant is important to the day-to-day safety of your client.

Character Trait 5 - You Must Be a Good Decision Maker

You've probably heard the old cliché' or expression, "It's better to be safe than sorry!" In the case of being a nursing assistant, it's ALWAYS best to go with safety first. The safety of your client, is always number one and if you are a person that abides by this rule, you will be absolutely fine.

There are many situations, which arise in providing day-to-day care to clients, which will demand of you to make good decisions. For example: Will this wheel chair fit through the door or do you need to use another safer entrance? Did they take their medications? Is the client ok to walk without a walker or do you need to give them the walker? Do you need to start using the gait belt with a client, because you've noticed weakness in their knees and legs and had to catch them several times? Do you need to get help before you perform a task? And the list goes on. But the main thing is always to remember, "It's better to be safe than sorry!"

Character Trait 6 - You Must Be a Good Listener

In providing care to clients, possessing good listening skills is a must. It requires that you listen not only for comprehension sake but you must also take into consideration any non-verbal communications. These non-verbal communications may take the form of facial expressions, nods, pointing and other bodily expressions. In my experience, I found that you will be communicated to in these ways a majority of the time.

Having good listening skills is also important when communicating with the client's primary care-giver (*the person that is solely responsible for the client—usually a relative*) and other health care personnel who provide care to the client. The information that you receive from them, will be indispensable in understanding your client's health condition, which will better equip you in properly providing care to the client.

Character Trait 7 - You Must Be a Dedicated Hard-Worker

Being a certified nursing assistant is not for everyone, because of the very nature of the job. It is a job that will require you to work, in many cases, 12-hour shifts (Day and Night)—3 to 4 days out of the week. Then on some occasions, you'll be asked to work overtime, due to someone calling in sick or late for work. Working these types of shifts can be draining and taxing on the body, especially if you are not used to working long hours. Yet in some instances you'll only work 8-hour shifts, nevertheless you'll need to be a hard worker.

Being a dedicated, hard-worker simple means that although you may be tired and weary, you must remain committed to providing quality service, practicing safe work habits, and at the same time maintain a caring and compassionate attitude.

Now, although breaks are necessary, you may not always be able to take breaks at your designated times due to unforeseeable emergency situations that will occur.

I'm reminded of an unforgettable incident that occurred, while I was doing my clinicals at a nursing home with a small group of nursing assistants. We had spent 4 hours with actual hands on experience, such as: taking vitals, transferring patients, providing perineal care, feeding, socializing, ambulation, etc., and it was nearing our time to leave. About this time me and another nursing assistant, were providing care to a female client that was on life-support and in a deep sleep.

What was about to happen took us by total surprise.

The woman flat-lined and died right before our eyes. The nurses rushed into the room and after they performed their vital checks and assessments, a confirmation of death was pronounced and the nursing assistants proceeded to clean the body.

The young lady that was working with me, burst into tears and we had to bring comfort to an uncomfortable and shocking situation, and we stayed there a lot longer than expected. Although this was a shocking and unforeseeable event that occurred, this was the reality of being a certified nursing assistant.

Conclusion

This is only a brief list of seven character traits, which I feel are important to possess, in order to become a successful nursing assistant. If you feel that you fit the bill then please continue reading. In the next chapter, I will be discussing what steps to take to become a certified nursing assistant.

Chapter 2 What are the Steps in Becoming a Certified Nursing Assistant?

"Faith is taking the first step even when you don't see the whole staircase. –Martin Luther King Jr."

The process of becoming a certified nursing assistant is not a difficult process, when you have the proper guidance and direction. The process can be broken down into the following:

- Visit your State Department of Health website to determine scope of practice
- Find schools in your area that are approved by your state
- Contact the schools or their website to get information on how to apply and ensure they are state-approved and you're comfortable with them
    - Find out if you will need to take a TB Skin test or Hepatitis shots, etc.
    - Find out the length of the program (*approx. 8-week/16-week*)
    - Find out the cost (*approx. $500-$1500*)
    - Find out do they offer day and evening classes
    - Find out what equipment you will need (*scrubs, stethoscope, etc.*)
    - Find out where the test site is located
    - Find out if they will assist you with employment upon completion of their program

- Download the certified nursing assistant State Handbook and the practice exams.
- Complete the program successfully
- Sign-up to take the state exam (*school should assist with this*)
- Take exam and pass both parts (written and skill) and obtain license
- Prepare for interview and apply for employment

This can be a daunting task, to try and complete all these steps on your own, therefore, we have done a majority of the leg work for you. All you have to do is visit our website at www.cnanationwide.com, and select your particular state and we will provide you with the following:

- Website link to your State Department of Health
- Website link to State Approved Schools with contact information
- Website link to download Nursing Assistant Handbook for your State.
- Website link to download practice exams for your written exam
- And much more…

If you have found the information on our site useful, then we ask that you please sign-up on our website and share this information with others.

Chapter 3. What Other Certifications are Required for Employment?

"I will study and prepare, and someday my opportunity will come.—Abraham Lincoln"

To land a job, in the Healthcare field as a certified nursing assistant, you must have completed a certified nursing assistant training program and obtained licensing by completing and passing the state written and skills exams. This would be considered the bare minimum job qualifications for employment as a certified nursing assistant. Although this is considered the bare minimum in qualifying for employment, many places of employment require further certifications.

So, what are these certifications?

In my research and experience, I found that most places require you to be certified in at least one or two of the following: First Aid, CPR, BLS (Basic Life Support), Phlebotomy, AED and EKG and in some special cases, for instance if you are working in Dialysis, you will be required in most states to obtain BONENT (Board of Nephrology Examiners Nursing and Technology) certifications. These requirements are all dependent on the facilities policies.

In some places of employment, they provide the extra necessary training once you are hired in. For example, they may provide CPR training free of charge once you are hired in. Then in other cases they may give you a designated amount of time, after you're hired in, to get the necessary certifications. For example, you could be given 6 months to obtain your BLS (Basic Life Support) training, while you are employed.

We will momentarily take a look at these certifications and discuss what they consist of and what you can expect. But just a word of caution, if you decide to take any of these certifications, many facilities require that the certification program be approved through the American Heart Association (AHA) and in some cases they require you to actually receive your training onsite, hands on and not online. So check with the certification program to ensure they are approved by the American Heart Association and that you read carefully the job posting requirements.

If you decide to take any of the following certifications, in which we will discuss below and cost is an issue, you'll be relieved to know that most places that offer these certifications will give you the option to purchase "blended courses". These blended courses may consist of two, three or more certification classes bundled together at one low price, which is cheaper than buying them separately. For instance some certification blended courses could be: Adult First Aid/CPR/AED, or Adult and Pediatric First Aid/CPR/AED, etc.

These blended courses come in many varieties, so make sure you look at purchasing a blended course versus purchasing them individually, if you want to save money in the long term.

First Aid

First Aid is what I would consider the most basic of certifications that you could acquire.

First aid according to OSHA, refers to medical attention that is usually administered immediately after the injury occurs and at the location where it occurred. It often consists of a one-time, short-term treatment and requires little technology or training to administer. First aid can include cleaning minor cuts, scrapes, or scratches; treating a minor burn; applying bandages and dressings; the use of non-prescription medicine; draining blisters; removing debris from the eyes; massage; and drinking fluids to relieve heat stress. OSHA's revised recordkeeping rule, which went into effect January 1, 2002, does not require first aid cases to be documented. For example: A worker goes to the first-aid room and has a dressing applied to a minor cut by a registered nurse. Although the registered nurse is a health care professional, the employer does not have to report the accident because the worker simply received first aid[1].

You can take First Aid certification class in-person and demonstrate all the skills and receive your certification. You'll also have the option to take part of the class online by watching videos and taking a test and then taking the remainder of it in-person to demonstrate the skills and receive your certification. Either way will be acceptable, as long as the program is approved by the American Heart Association.

CPR

CPR, also known as Cardiopulmonary Resuscitation is a very important certification to obtain. It's a certification that's mandatory in a majority of medical facilities across the country.

Possessing this all-important skill and certification can truly be a lifesaving technique. Cardiopulmonary Resuscitation keeps oxygenated blood flowing throughout a person's body while preventing severe damage of tissues and keeping them alive long enough to receive professional medical attention.

According to the American Heart Association, about 92 percent of sudden cardiac arrest victims die before reaching the hospital, but statistics prove that if more people knew CPR, more lives could be saved. Immediate CPR can double, or even triple, a victim's chance of survival[2].

I've only seen this class being taught in-person, due to the importance of learning the CPR skills and techniques correctly.

When I took this class it was an eye-opening experience for me. I didn't realize of how strenuous and draining it can be to properly perform CPR in a life-threatening situation and this was only simulated training.

I would highly recommend that you take this class and obtain the certification.

Basic Life Support (BLS)

Above any course that I've mentioned thus far, BLS or Basic Life Support is the course that I would personally, highly recommend to take, because it was the most mentioned certification requirement in many of the job postings online for certified nursing assistants.

The Basic Life Support for Healthcare Providers is specifically designed to provide a broad variety of healthcare professionals the ability to recognize several life-threatening emergencies and to provide CPR, use an AED (Automated External Defibrillator), and relieve choking victims in a safe, timely and effective manner. This course acts as a combination course or what most people refer to as blended courses, that puts CPR, AED and the relieving of choking victims together, which makes it a great course and money-saving deal that will save you money and time and if you were to try and take them separately.

In the Basic Life Support class you will learn the critical concepts of CPR, The American Heart Association Chain of Survival, 1-Rescuer CPR and AED for adult, child and infant, 2-Rescurer CPR and AED for adult, child and infant, Bag-mask techniques, Rescue breathing and Relief of choking victims[3].

You can also take the ACLS otherwise known as Advanced Cardiovascular Life Support, if you decide to further your knowledge in the Life Support area. Most instructors that I've talked with recommended it, but I haven't seen it being a requirement for employment as a certified nursing assistant.

Phlebotomy and EKG

Taking Phlebotomy and EKG, is heavily dependent on what state you are in. Some states allow certified nursing assistants to draw blood and other states do not. But if you will be working at a facility, in which it is lawful, then you must have the phlebotomy certification.

If you are planning to become a Patient Care Technician, which is slightly more advanced, in some cases, to the certified nursing assistant, then you will likely have to take this advanced course along with EKG. This will vary depending on what state you are in.

Advice on Deciding Which Certifications to Take

Read through the job qualifications sections of job postings in your area to get a general idea of what certifications are required. If you find that a majority of jobs listed, require a particular certification, then it will be best to go ahead and get that particular certification, so that you will be prepared and to broaden your list of potential places of employment.

Conclusion

Should you obtain these certifications is something you must decide, but obtaining at least one to two of these certifications is beneficial in meeting the qualifications for employment, making your applications stand out, potentially increasing your starting salary and expanding your knowledge base in the Healthcare field.

Also if you decide to take any of these certifications, make sure to keep them updated as they will expire, especially your certified nursing assistant license. When I was receiving my training to become a certified nursing assistant, a lady in our class warned us of this because she had let her license expire and had to retake the entire certified nursing assistant program over and the state and skills exam before she could receive her license. This cost her a lot of unnecessary time and money, so don't let this happen to you.

Chapter 4. What are the Different Areas That a Certified Nursing Assistant Can Work?

"Everyone enjoys doing the kind of work for which he is best suited." – Napoleon Hill

In working in the Healthcare field as a certified nursing assistant, you'll be working under the direct supervision of a nurse, which could be a LPN/LVN (*Licensed Practical Nurse/Licensed Vocational Nurse*) or a RN (*Registered Nurse*). Under their supervision and direction you will typically provide assistance by administering general care such as: bathing, dressing, feeding, toileting, oral care, transferring, ambulation and taking of vital signs such as: temperature, blood pressure, pulse and respiration and reporting any significant changes of condition of your patients to the nurses.

As a nursing assistant you are considered to be the backbone or major support on the healthcare team. The nurses depend heavily on certified nursing assistants, so that they are free to do their jobs.

The most well-known areas where certified nursing assistants work in, are long term care facilities (*nursing homes*) and Home Health Care Agencies. Although these are the main two areas, the following are other areas that hire certified nursing assistants:

- Assisted Living Facilities
- Staffing Agencies
- Hospitals
- Hospices
- Adult Day Care

So what area should you work in?

In the next section, I will be discussing the pros and cons of working in the various afore mentioned places, such that you will be able to make a more informed decision on what area would be more suitable for you.

Nursing Homes

Nursing Homes, also referred to as: Long Term Care Centers, Skilled Nursing Facilities, Care Homes or Rest Homes, houses the elderly and adults with physical and/or mental disabilities[1,] where skilled nurses and certified nursing assistants provide personal or nursing care 24 hours/7 days a week.[2.] Along with the nursing care, most facilities also provide physical therapy, speech therapy and occupational therapy.

Nursing Homes are intended for people that don't need to be hospitalized but can't be cared for properly at home, therefore, the nursing home becomes their new home or place of residency and they are referred to as residents and not patients and are made to feel at home as much as possible.

I personally enjoyed working in a nursing home and it's a great place to gain lots of valuable experience, especially if you're interested in furthering your career to become a LPN or RN.

Pros:
- Working primarily with the elderly
- Gain lots of experience
- Work close with nurses and other therapists
- Family type environment
- Daily routine
- Room for advancement
- Less stressful
- Tuition reimbursement
- Great preparation for becoming a LPN\LVN or RN

Cons:
- Understaffed situations
- Lots of paperwork
- Burnout
- Long shifts

Assisted Living Facilities

Assisted Living is a great option for many older people that are entering into their senior years. Assisted Living Communities, provides senior adults, who can live independently, with whatever assistance they need, that would help them to live out their lives to the fullest.

They provide services such as: 24-hour supervision and security, daily meals, basic housekeeping, laundry, health and exercise programs, transportation and daily activities and care. This is where the certified nursing assistant job comes in and that is to provide the clients with what we call ADL or Activities of Daily Living such as: dressing, eating, mobility, hygiene, bathing, toileting, using the telephone, shopping, etc.

Pros:
- Set your own work schedule
- Not as stressful

Cons:
- Caring for clients that need too much care and needs to be in a nursing home
- Understaffed
- Work overload

Staffing Agencies

Once you complete your Nursing Assistant Training Program and become certified, joining a staffing agency can be a good place to start, while you are looking for permanent employment, but it comes with its own unique set of pros and cons, especially for someone just starting out in this field, in which we will cover shortly.

Nursing Agencies also referred to as Nursing Registry, are numerous all across the nation. They provide registered nurses, licensed practical nurses, certified nursing assistants, home health aides, and companions with short-term job opportunities in their respected fields, which may lead to permanent jobs. These jobs are found in a multitude of healthcare facilities such as: Hospitals, Medical Offices, Nursing Homes, private care, etc[3]. The need arises for capable certified nursing assistants in facilities due to reasons such as: understaffing, during vacationing months, holidays, etc.

Although this seems like a good place to start, especially when you are just starting out and putting in resumes to find permanent work, yet it may not be, for several reasons.

The first being that if you are assigned to work at a facility, the expectation will be to get right to work in most cases (*most nursing assistants refer to this as being thrown to the wolves*), with no training or orientation; therefore you must be capable of performing basic skills and be able to professionally adapt to any situation. Therefore, if you lack in the area of experience, you won't be able to do your job with confidence and you may require lots of help, which may make an impression to the facility that you don't know what you are doing which could hurt you from receiving any future assignments. My advice is to be totally transparent and honest, in explaining to them you may need some temporary assistance.

But once you gain more experience as a certified nursing assistant, and you need a way to supplement your income and at the same time gain some valuable experience in various areas of the Healthcare Field, this would be an opportunity to take advantage of because you can work as many hours as needed and not be under any obligations.

Pros:
- Flexible scheduling
- Experience in various types of Healthcare facilities
- Resume building experience
- Meeting lots of different people and Healthcare Professionals
- Potential opportunities for permanent employment
- Great preparation for becoming a LPN\LVN or RN

Cons:
- No definite amount of work
- Little or no orientation or training upon accepting an assignment
- Short-term assignments
- Assignments being cancelled

Hospitals

Hospitals are arguably the best and most well-known areas to work in, as certified nursing assistants. Hospital jobs are the best jobs overall, due to better medical benefits, greater pay, tuition reimbursement, larger health support systems, varied work experience and many areas for potential advancement.

It's also a great place to work due to the experience and knowledge gained from working alongside other health care professionals such as: Doctors, Nurses, Occupational Therapist, Physical Therapists, Speech Therapist, etc. This experience is invaluable, if you have plans on furthering your career, to become a Registered Nurse, Licensed Practical Nurse, or any other Healthcare professional such as a Physical Therapist, Occupational Therapist, Paramedic, etc.

Landing a job at a hospital can be somewhat of a difficult task because of the hiring process. Most of the hospitals that I've visited or worked at, offer job opportunities internally first and then after a certain expiration date, to the general public. This is great news if you are already employed at a hospital and want to find employment as a certified nursing assistant, but if you are not, then the harder it will be to get a job there.

Here are few suggestions if you are in this situation:

1. Volunteer at the hospital in which you would like to work. This will allow you to demonstrate yourself, your work ethic and initiative to those that are responsible in the hiring process.
2. Have someone on the inside, who can vouch for your character and work ethic to help you get an interview.

Pros:
- Medical Benefits (Dental, Vision, etc.)
- Higher wages
- Tuition reimbursement
- Larger Health Support Teams
- Gain experience in lots of areas
- Potential for advancement to other areas within the Hospital

Cons:
- Difficulty getting hired

Home Health Agency

One of the most familiar provider of home care services is that of the Home Health Agency. The primary purpose of this type of agency is to provide skilled care for treatment or rehabilitation services to homebound patients. These services include skilled nursing, physical and occupational therapy, social work and home health aide, while under professional supervision. A non-medical home care agency is an agency that provides home care services although they are not considered to be skilled care. The types of agencies provide what is labelled as non-skilled supportive custodial care that is supplied by home health aides, certified nursing assistants (CNAs) and also noncertified nurse aides, homemakers, and companions[4].

In my opinion and through my own personal work experience, working for a Home Health Aide Agency is one of the best jobs for a certified nursing assistant. Unlike working for a Nursing Home or hospital, where you are responsible for 8-12 patients or more, you'll only be caring for one patient at a time, where you will travel to their home or place of residency and provide care, for about 4-12 hours a day, depending on the client's individual needs. Although you will only be working with one client at a time, you may be assigned 1-3 clients. You'll provide services such as bathing, dressing, toileting, eating and providing transportation to medical appointments, grocery stores, and recreational activities.

Once you are hired on with a Home Health Agency, in most cases, the agency will assign you to 1 to 2 clients, where you will meet-and-greet with the client and their primary caregiver and go through a mini-interview. If the primary care giver approves of you then they will contact the Agency and you'll start working with that particular client and providing care. Otherwise, the Agency will continue to try and connect you with the right clients. Due to this process, it may take a while to be on a consistent work schedule.

Pros:

- Working with only one client at a time
- Flexible scheduling
- Less stressful
- Availability of various shifts, 4-24 hours
- Payment for mileage when transporting clients

Cons:

- Clients may have to be moved to skilled nursing home
- Clients may pass away

Hospice Care

A hospice is defined as a medical facility providing emotional and mental health care services for patients who are terminally ill along with their families. A certified nursing assistant that takes a job in Hospice Care is referred to as a Hospice CNA, where they will either work in a facility or a patient's home.

Deciding to become a Hospice CNA is not something to be taken lightly, due to the nature of the job. As a Hospice CNA you will be responsible for meeting the patient general needs such as: changing bed linens, assisting with transportation, bathing patients, transferring from beds to wheelchairs, maintaining accurate and confidential records regarding each patient, preparing meals, checking various vital signs, performing duties requested by clients and families, assisting with exercise, administering medications, and changing dressings.

On top of these responsibilities, you will also be responsible for providing emotional support for the clients and their family members. Therefore, you must be able to demonstrate a strong, patient and compassionate attitude during service and possess resilient bedside manners and remain calm under pressure and have the ability to teach the family how to provide certain types of care to their loved ones.

Most of all you must be able to handle the dying of a patient in your presence. This can be really tough for some people and easy for others. So if you have a difficult time with death, then this may not be for you. You must also be comfortable with cleaning and preparing a dead body and comforting the family. This I can say is not for everyone.

A certified nursing assistant that chooses this area to work in, needs to be a nursing assistant with several years of experience, who's strong enough to handle death and all it entails and skilled enough to provide great care to the client and also able to teach the family and console them in their time of need.

Pros:
- Pay rate is a lot higher than other areas of employment for CNAs

Cons:
- Demanding and stressful
- Very emotional
- Long hours
- Experiencing death often

Adult Day Care

Adult Day Care is a great health care option for many primary care givers who have elderly loved ones who need around the clock care, especially during the day when the care giver must work due to financial responsibilities. This also gives the primary care giver much needed rest and relaxation, time to handle personal business and at the same time it gives them a sense of peace of mind knowing that their loved ones are receiving great care in a friendly environment. It also provides the older adult with an opportunity to get out of the house and receive both mental and social stimulation.

Adult Day Care facilities provide a wide range of care such as: personal care, therapeutic activities, nursing care, and meals such as breakfast, lunch and snacks. They also provide various activities and services such as:

- Audiology
- Counseling
- Exercise Classes
- Hair and Beauty Services
- Massage Therapy
- Occupational Therapy
- Companionship
- Medical Care
- Socialization
- Transportation

The staff at an Adult Day Care Facility usually consist of a center director, social worker, an activity director, registered or licensed practical nurse and experienced certified nursing assistants. The certified nursing assistants in the Adult Day Care provides short-term daily care for physically or mentally impaired adults, where the level of care will be different, depending on the type of care needed.

Pros:
- Great pay
- Day shift work
- Working with different types of clients to gain experience

Cons:
- Most require at least one year of experience as a CNA.

Chapter 5. What is the Job Outlook and Pay Rate for Certified Nursing Assistants?

"Life…It tends to respond to our outlook, to shape itself to meet our expectations." –
Richard M. Devos

What Do the Statistics Tell Us?

The Job outlook for certified nursing assistant looks strong due to the high demand for healthcare in an increasingly growing elderly population particularly in the baby boomer population. It is estimated according to the Administration on Aging, that the 65 years and older population will see an increase in the years 2010 to 2050, going from 40,229,000 to 88,547,000 in the United States alone[1].

This increase in the elderly population over the next few decades, will have a positive effect in the HealthCare field by opening up the HealthCare field with many job opportunities, especially in the area of Nursing (RNs/LPNs/certified nursing assistants/orderlies).

Job growth for nursing assistants and orderlies is expected to grow 17% from 2014 to 2024, according to the United States Bureau of Labor Statistics[2]. This growth rate is faster than the average for all occupations[2]. See chart below.

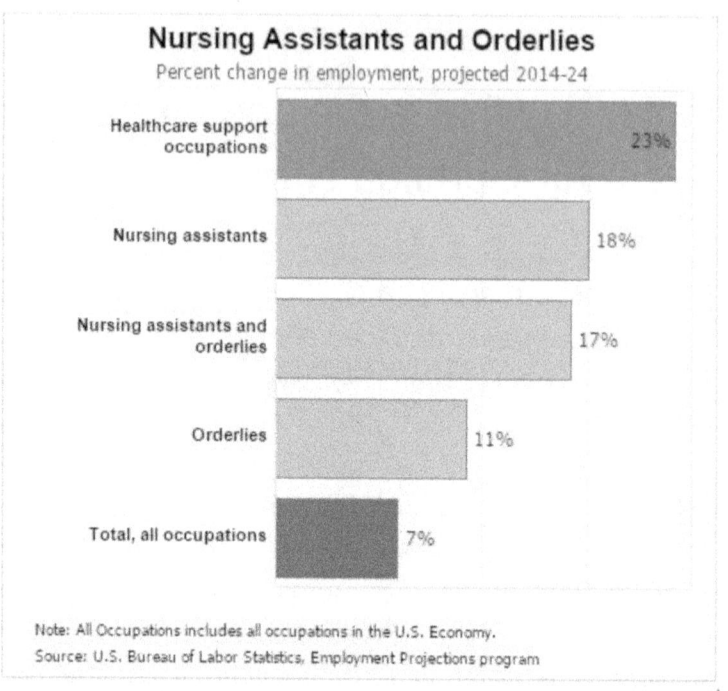

Nursing Assistants and Orderlies

Percent change in employment, projected 2014-24

Occupation	Percent
Healthcare support occupations	23%
Nursing assistants	18%
Nursing assistants and orderlies	17%
Orderlies	11%
Total, all occupations	7%

Note: All Occupations includes all occupations in the U.S. Economy.
Source: U.S. Bureau of Labor Statistics, Employment Projections program

These statistics are quite impressive to say the least. So if there were any doubts in your mind of how reliable the future job market would be for certified nursing assistants, then hopefully these statistics will resolve any of your doubts.

To add to the above statistics is the fact that, for nursing assistants who have completed a state-approved educational training program, and obtained their licensing by passing their written and skill exam, can expect the employment projections for them to steadily increase. According to the United States Bureau of Labor Statistics, Employment Projections Data for nursing assistants and orderlies, 2014-24, will see an increase in employment going from 1,492,400 to 1,754,100 for nursing assistants and 53,000 to 58,800 for orderlies.[3]

The statistics so far is favorable towards becoming a certified nursing assistant with the exception that with the increasing number of baby boomers retiring and using government based programs such as Medicare and Medicaid, may cause unwanted cuts to the program which may affect their ability to pay for nursing home care, because nursing home care can be expensive. Just to give you an idea of the cost, according to LongTermCare.gov[4] they list the estimated cost of Long Term Care as Follows:

Some average costs for long-term care in the United States (in 2010) were:

- $205 per day or $6,235 per month for a semi-private room in a nursing home
- $229 per day or $6,965 per month for a private room in a nursing home
- $3,293 per month for care in an assisted living facility (for a one-bedroom unit)
- $21 per hour for a home health aide
- $19 per hour for homemaker services
- $67 per day for services in an adult day health care center

In addition to the cuts that may occur to Medicare and Medicaid, federal and state funding are increasing the demand for home and community-based long-term care, which saves money and also leads to more opportunities for certified nursing assistants working in home health and community rehabilitation services.

What is the Pay Rate for Certified Nursing Assistants

The pay rate of certified nursing assistants according to *Payscale.com*[5], put earnings between $18,385 and $31,672 a year as of September 2015, where the median salary was $24,245. The median wage refers to the wage "in the middle." Which means half the workers earned below this level.

The pay rate of certified nursing assistants varies due to factors such as: experience, state of employment, skills and type of industry. If you have 5 to 10 years of experience, and have a large skill set then you'll probably be able to better negotiate higher pay than someone with less than 5 years of experience and a lesser skill set. The pay rate is also heavily dependent upon the state in which you'll be working in. The diagram[6] below shows the annual mean wage of nursing assistants, by state as of May 2014:

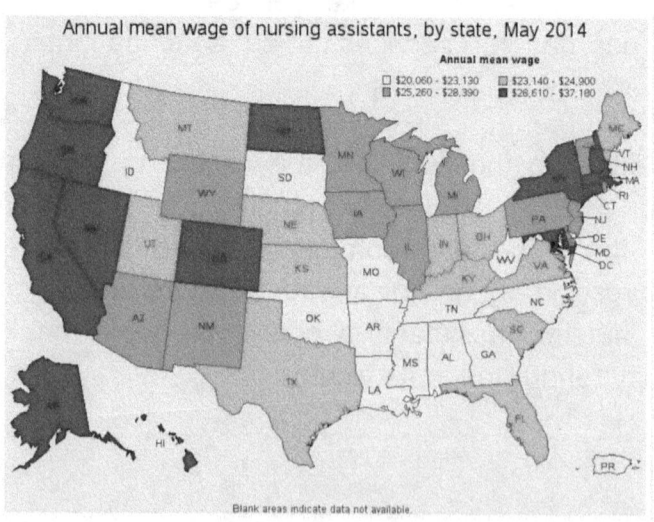

Annual mean wage of nursing assistants, by state, May 2014

Blank areas indicate data not available.

The last important factor that will contribute to determining pay rate, is the industry in which you will work. According to the 2014, United States Bureau of Labor Statistics the following area have the following median annual wages:

Annual Media Wage 2014—Bureau of Labor Statistics[7]	
Government	$30,200
Hospitals; state, local , and private	27,360
Nursing Care Facilities(skilled)	24,120
Continuing Care Retirement Communities and assisted living facilities for the elderly	23,650
Home Healthcare Services	23,080

After examining all the pay rates in the above table, you must personally decide what area you would enjoy working in. If money is the bottom line for you then it would be better to go with Government or Hospital jobs, but if you are you planning to advance further in your career to a LPN, RN or any other Healthcare medical position, then keep in mind that the experience you gain in certain jobs will be key in preparing you for more advanced careers. The career path for a certified nursing assistant can be as follows[8]:

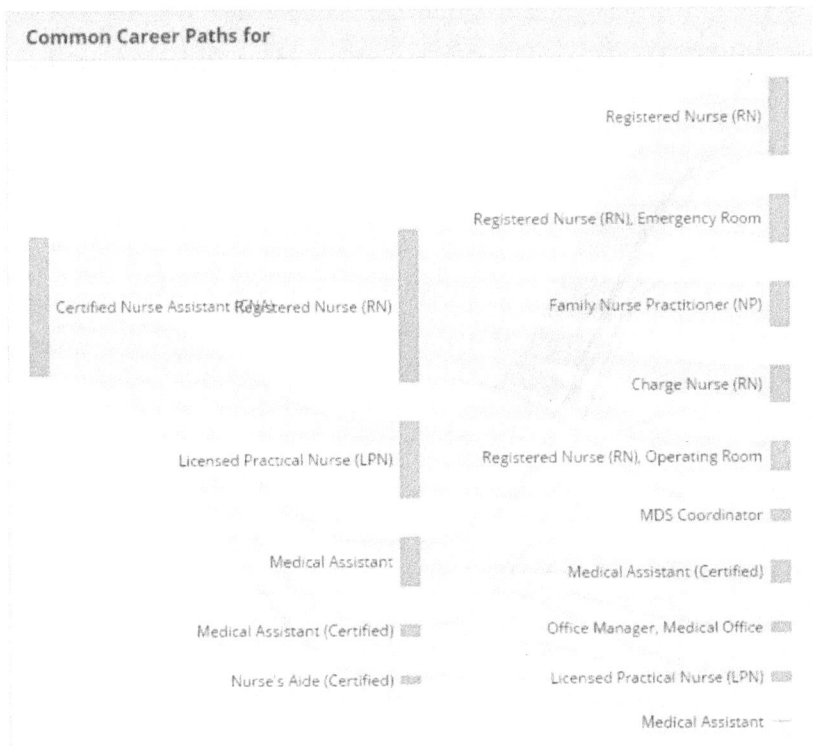

Conclusion

In conclusion, becoming a certified nursing assistant can be a great and rewarding career in many ways and can also be a stepping stone to more advanced medical careers. As a career, you'll have the satisfaction of knowing that you are improving the quality of someone's life by assisting them in their daily living activities and providing them with safety thereby helping them to feel more secure in an unsecure world. As a stepping stone, it will allow you to move on to more advanced positions in the medical field, thereby increasing your skill set and salary.

Chapter 6. Interview Tips

"You've got to believe deep inside yourself that you're destined to do great things." –
Joe Paterno

Once you have successfully completed your state-approved training program and passed the written and skilled exams and obtained your license, the next big step in the process is applying for jobs and preparing for interviews. This whole process of searching for jobs, putting in resumes and preparing for interviews can be a stressful and tedious process, therefore, it will be necessary to be thoroughly prepared.

In Chapters 4 and 5, I've provided lots of relative information that will help guide you in the process of selecting a job that would be suitable for you, therefore, in this chapter, I would like to focus on preparing for the interview, which is the most critical part of the process. If you get this part right, you'll greatly increase your chances of getting hired in the job that you so desire.

So the question is how do you successfully prepare for the interview?

Understanding the Purpose of the Interview

One of the first things to understand about an interview is its purpose, which is two-fold.

The purpose of an interview, from the interviewer's perspective is to see if you fit the criteria of particular position that needs to be filled in their company—period. So, it is important that you know exactly what it is they are looking for. For example are they looking for a specific set of traits, such as: compassion, empathy, caring, initiator, or are there a certain set of skills they are looking for, such as: nursing skills, teamwork, organizational skills, etc.

Secondly, the purpose of an interview from the interviewee's (*your*) perspective is to convince the interviewer, that you are the person they are looking for. This is accomplished by having clear and thorough examples of how you successfully demonstrated the traits and skills that they are looking for.

So how do you accomplish this?

Preparation for Using the S.T.A.R. System

In the next section, I will be discussing the S.T.A.R. System that will help guide you in preparing for your interview by being able to thoroughly convince the interviewer that you are the person they are looking for, by providing clear examples on how you have the skills and traits they are looking for, but before I discuss this system I would like to lay some important ground work.

Before using this system, you will need to read and re-read the job posting's criteria and get a clear and thorough understanding of what it is they are looking for. Write these things down on a piece of paper, underline or highlight them. Next, write down, out beside each criteria, examples of how you can prove, or demonstrate this criteria. In the table below, I've provided a brief example:

Job Posting: Looking to hire <u>compassionate certified nursing assistant</u> with <u>1-2 years of experience</u>, with <u>great organizational skills</u>.	
Compassionate	Examples: Took care of elderly lady in community, volunteered at nursing home, etc.
Certified nursing assistant	Copy of certified nursing licenses that are up-to-date
1-2 years of experience	Nursing home – Shady Oaks (2 years).
Great organizational skills	Responsible at Shady Oaks to make out bathing schedules for all clients in the facility.

Now as you can see that some of the criteria are quite easy to prove and provide evidence for, such as your certified nursing assistant licenses and the 1-2 years of experience, but with the character traits and skills (*Compassionate and Great organizational skills*) you'll need specific examples (*as many as you like, the more the better-trust me*) to prove you are compassionate and possess great organizational skills.

In the next section, I will show you how to develop and present these specific examples to the interviewer that will have impact, make a lasting impression and help you to stand out amongst the competition.

Using the S.T.A.R System in the Interview

The S.T.A.R. system is a system used and taught at Toyota Motor Manufacturing. Although the S.T.A.R. system is used predominately in the preparation and presentation of various types of projects and activities within Toyota, it is also used in preparing for interviews.

The S.T.A.R. system, stands for Situation, Task, Action and Results.

- Situation: This is an example of what we are trying to prove.
- Task: This is what we needed to do.
- Action: This is what we did.
- Results: This was the end results of what we did.

Now that we know what the S.T.A.R. system means, let's now apply it to the interview process.

In the previous sections we wrote down, highlighted or underlined those specific criteria that the company was looking for in its applicants. The criteria that we needed to be able to prove with examples involved traits and skills. In the following example below, we will look at a trait that is part of the criteria and provide proof for that trait using the S.T.A.R. system.

Question by Interviewer: Tell us about yourself? (*They are looking to hire someone that is compassionate*)

Answer: I consider myself to be a <u>compassionate</u> person that looks on the needs of others and tries to meet those needs.

Situation – I remember a situation when I was working with an elderly lady that had an operation on her hip and she wasn't able to cook or clean her home.

Task –So I thought how could I provide assistance until she is healed and able again?

Action –I went to her home, I prepared her meals for breakfast, lunch and dinner. I also set a picture of ice water with several snacks and fruit by her bedside in case she got hungry. I did this for about 3 months, until she was healed enough to do things on her own.

Results –Her attitude and quality of life was improved greatly and she responded by writing me a letter and thanking me for helping her and gave me a check for $300.00.

If you use this system on every question that is asked and on the ones you think you may be asked, you'll do very well in an interview. But make sure to have lots of examples, and remember the acronym, S.T.A.R – Situation, Task, Action and Result.

What are Some of the Questions That You May Be Asked?

I've listed below some common questions that you may be asked during an interview, along with some tips. Make sure to use the S.T.A.R. system, when answering them.

Question 1: Can you tell me a little about yourself?
Tip –The interviewer is using this question to find out how well you will make a good certified nursing assistant. So don't focus or talk on unrelated things that don't pertain to the job. Instead focus on what they are looking for. That's the part of "You" that they are interested in. So discuss using the S.T.A.R. system on how your experiences and personality would make you a good certified nursing assistant.

Question 2: Why do you want to work as a certified nursing assistant?
Tip —The interviewer is using this question to assess your passion for working in the medical field. So anything that you did medically, prior to becoming a certified nursing assistant would be helpful. It can be just as simply as you volunteered in Nursing Homes, or you took care of a love one, etc. Just make sure to use the S.T.A.R system so that you'll be able to paint a clear and vivid picture of your passion.

Question 3: Why did you leave your last job?
Tip –The key here and with all the questions is to stay positive. Don't go into any negative situations, they will only lessen your chances of landing a job. Just mention positive things that you learned on your previous job and how this career change is more akin to your talents and skills.

Question 4: Where do you want to be 5 years from now?
Tip – I can say hands down if you answer this question correctly, you'll get great points in landing a job. So sit down and actually plan out, where you would want to be. If you desire to further your career by becoming a Medical Assistant, LPN or RN then be able to explain, while at the same time expressing how working at a reputable company, you would be able to gain invaluable experience and to learn from some of the best in the business that provide outstanding and quality care to clients.

Question 5: What is your greatest strength?
Tip – If you get asked this question, then this is the time you can really shine with an answer. Because the medical field is really demanding in the area of possessing great organizational skills, being prompt and on time, or being able to operate under pressure. If you have any of these three particular strengths, then by all means be prepared to express them and give examples.

Question 6: What were your grades?
Tip – It's best to bring a copy of your transcript to the interview of the school that you attended in receiving your nursing assistant training. This will give the interviewer a snap-shot view of how serious you consider your career as a certified nursing assistant.

Question 7: How would you deal with difficult patients?
Tip – There are two key elements in successfully answering this question and they are what is your attitude during this difficult situation and how do you problem-solve the difficulty. You want to first express to the interviewer, that you have the ability to remain calm and under control in difficult situations. Secondly, you need to be able to express your problem

solving skills. I learned an invaluable problem solving skill, which I would like to share with you. It's called the 5 why's of problem solving and it will help you get to the root cause of any problem. I've included a diagram on the next page along with an example:

The Five Why's of Problem Solving Situation:

Why: _____?

Why: _____?

Why: _____?

Why: _____?

Why: (Root Cause) _____?

Example: Let's say for instance, you had a difficult situation, in working with an elderly man that fussed and fought, every time someone tried to transfer him from the bed to his wheel chair. How would you handle this? The first thing is to remain calm and try and calm the client down, while maintaining low and gentle tones. Secondly, is to use the problem solving skill above to get to the root of why the client fusses and fights when he is transferred to his wheel chair.

Situation: Client Fusses and fights during transfer to wheel chair
Why: Client doesn't like wheel chair
  Why: The Chair is uncomfortable
    Why: The Chair has tears and rips and exposed metal that cuts client
    Why: The Chair is out of commissioned, but isn't labelled and is still being used
      Why: (Root Cause) Maintenance forgot to label and take off floor.

Now as you can readily see, there was a legitimate reasoning behind this difficult situation, where the root cause we found to be—Maintenance forgot to label the chair as an out of commissioned chair and take it off the floor. Now, if you hadn't went through this problem solving technique, you could have mistakenly placed the problem on the client instead of Maintenance.

I hope you can see how powerful this problem solving technique is, when trying to get the root of problems.

To see if your Problem solving make sense and correct, start with the root cause and traverse the 5 why's by using the word "therefore". If done correctly it should make perfect sense, otherwise you should redo it until it makes sense.

For example:
Maintenance forgot to label the chair as out-of-commission and take off floor
THEREFORE
The chair is out-of-commissioned and isn't labelled and is being used
THERFORE
The chair has tears, rips and exposed metal that cuts the client
THERFORE
The chair is uncomfortable
THERFORE
The Client doesn't likes the chair
THEREFORE
The Client fusses and fights during transfer to the wheel chair.

You won't necessarily always have 5 why's. You may have fewer or more, but 5 is usually ideal. Just expressing to the interviewer that you have a process of problem-solving will be impressive to say the least.

Conclusion

In conclusion you must be mindful of the fact, that the most important thing to clearly communicate to your employer is that you have a strong passion and desire for helping others and that you present yourself confidently, friendly and knowledgeable. This will all greatly increase your chances of being hired.

Chapter 7. Advancing in Your Career

"I'm looking forward to the future, and feeling grateful for the past" – Mike Rowe

Certified Nursing Assistant as a Career Choice

Choosing to be a certified nursing assistant, as a career choice, is a decision that many people make. They find it a great joy, to provide quality care and services to their clients and wouldn't be happier doing anything else. This provides them with a deep sense of satisfaction in knowing that they are making a positive difference in someone else's life.

Along with the opportunity of improving the quality of someone else's life, the opportunity to increase one's personal knowledge in the Healthcare field is offered by taking continuing education courses, attending seminars and various workshops and joining community-based organizations that cater to Primary Care Givers. Some such organizations to join is the American Caregiver Association (**https://www.americancaregiverassociation.org**) or the National Association for Home Care & Hospice (NAHC) **http://www.nahc.org**.

So, there will always be ample room for continued learning and growth in the Healthcare field as a career oriented certified nursing assistant.

Becoming a Self-employed Certified Nursing Assistant

Due to the very low wages that are paid to certified nursing assistants, many choose to become self-employed to increase their income, thereby improving the quality of their life. This option should only be chosen once you have at least 2-3 years of experience as a certified nursing assistant. Although this 2-3 years of experience is not mandatory, it will provide you with the confidence and much needed experience to enable you to provide quality care and services to your clients and to make you and your business more marketable.

Why is now the best time to consider this option?

With the increased amount of seniors—especially the baby boomers retiring soon, this will place a demand in the market for reputable self-employed certified nursing assistants, who are trustworthy and that can provide high quality services at an affordable price, which will save retirees thousands of dollars in cost, if they decide to live in their homes and receive this type of care.

So how do you get started in becoming a self-employed independent contractor—certified nursing assistant?

The first step will be to ensure that you have obtained the basic things, such as: up-to-date CNA licenses, BLS (Basic Life Support) and/or First Aid certifications, TB shot, and a list of references and work experience (_If you are currently employed as a CNA then you may already have most of these things_).

Why are these things important?

The family or another individual overseeing the care of their loved one is likely to be skeptical about your qualifications and abilities, if you don't possess these things such as licenses, First Aid certifications, references, etc. These things will provide you with the credibility you need to present yourself as a qualified and competent caregiver.

Once you have the basic things covered the next step is to get a general idea of what type of clients you would like to work with and what type of services you'll be providing. Do you want to work only with children with disabilities? Do you want to work with elderly women only—that's fairly independent? Do you want to work with seniors—men or women that are very dependent? Do you want to work with disabled veterans, and the list goes on. The following is a brief list of the services that you can provide:

- Cooking meals
- Laundry
- Light House Cleaning
- Grocery Shopping
- Companionship
- Assisting with Activities of Daily Living such as: combing/washing hair, brushing teeth, bathing/showering, dressing, exercises, etc.

This is an important step in the process for a number of reasons. The first being, you'll be creating a niche market for your business—a business that's focused in on providing services and care to only a particular group of people. This will help steer you away from jobs that you've already decided, you are not particularly interested in. Secondly, it will help by keeping your pricing, services and care fairly consistent from one customer to the next. Thirdly, it will help you in marketing and getting business to customers that are looking for caregivers in your particular niche.

After you have determined your niche then you will need to determine, how much to charge. This can be somewhat of a difficult step in the process, because you don't want to overcharge nor do you want to undercharge. The general rate is somewhere, between, $10.00 and $20.00 per hour. Also make sure to include transportation fees if you will be using your own vehicle, usually about .50/mile is a reasonable rate.

The next step is to register with Medicare and Medicaid services board to be a licensed independent service provider. They may require that you take additional classes to ensure that you understand their rules and regulations. However, after becoming registered, you'll be able to work for government agencies, specialty agencies or anyone who uses Medicare/Medicaid type insurance. You also have the option to seek out clients on your own, in building your clientele.

Next, you will need to check with your local city or county division of licensing to determine what type of license you need for your business. Once you get your business license, you'll need to look into obtaining bonding, insurance and consider getting a LLC (Limited Liability Company) (*A LLC provides protection for your business, LegalZoom* (**https://www.legalzoom.com**) *is an affordable option*).

This is only a basic plan to starting your business, but keep in mind to check with your local city and county division for all the legal information in starting your business, because laws differ from state to state.

Certified Nursing Assistant as a Doorway to More Advanced Medical Careers

Many licensed practical nurses and registered nurses, started their careers out as certified nursing assistants and it has been testified that the knowledge and experience gained from being a certified nursing assistant, prior to becoming a LPN or RN, is to go without saying—invaluable and indispensable.

I've compiled a list of the benefits of being a certified nursing assistant prior to progressing to further more advanced medical careers as follows:

- You'll know inwardly if this field of nursing is right for you or not.
- You'll learn the very basic principles of nursing.
- You'll learn from hands on experience.
- You'll have the opportunity to work with other Healthcare Team Members—doctors, nurses, physical therapists, occupational therapists, nutritionist, etc.
- You'll become acquainted with medical terminology.
- You'll learn how to operate various medical machinery and equipment such as—Hoyer Lifts, Standing Lifts, hospital beds, blood pressure/pulse/temperature machines, stethoscopes, thermometers, etc.
- You'll have the opportunity to take classes offered through your employer, which are usually free or cost a small fee.
- You'll be more advanced than a person that's pursuing a nursing degree with no prior work experience.
- You'll be able to increase your chances of a higher salary due to your prior work experience.

Although this is a small list, I've endeavored to highlight the major benefits of becoming a certified nursing assistant before advancing to more advanced careers.

Once you have gained experience from being a certified nursing assistant and you wish to further your career in the nursing field, then you are faced with a new set of questions:

Do I become a LPN first? Do I go for 2 years and get RN (A.D.N.)? Do I go 4 years and get RN (B.S.N.)?

In the next chapter, "Choosing a Nursing Path—LPN or RN", I'll be discussing on making this important decision further.

Chapter 8. Choosing a Nursing Path— LPN or RN

Choosing to advance in your career by becoming a licensed practical nurse or a registered nurse is a wise decision. Wise in that you will be advancing in the Healthcare field by broadening your knowledge base, taking upon greater responsibilities and being rewarded with an increase in salary.

So the question is, "Do you want to become a licensed practical nurse or a registered nurse?"

I've personally done research online and by talking with LPNs and RNs and even CNAs that were in school to become LPNs and RNs, all their answers varied. Some suggested it was better to become a LPN first, while others suggested it would be better to attend a 2-year school to become a RN (A.D.N.) and while others suggested to attend 4 years to get the RN (B.S.N.) degree.

So who's right?

From my perspective they were all right, in the sense that what they choose, they choose, because it was what was BEST for THEM. And this is the way that you must choose, after examining your options thoroughly, is what is BEST for YOU.

Listed below is a brief description of the licensed practical nurse and the registered nurse.

Licensed Practical Nurse Job Description

Licensed practical nurses work under the direct supervision of registered nurses and physicians. In the United States, licensed practical nurses are also referred to as LVNs (*licensed vocational nurses*) in the states of California and Texas. However, in the Canadian province of Ontario, they are referred to as RPNs (*registered practical nurses*).

The job of a licensed practical nurse or licensed vocational nurse involves the following:

- Provide basic bedside care
- Maintaining records of patients' histories
- Provide dressing or bathing assistance
- Update doctors and registered nurses on a patient's status
- Measure vital signs such as weight, height, temperature, blood pressure, pulse and respiratory rate
- Assist doctors and registered nurses with tests and procedures
- Caring for and feeding infants
- Assemble, use and clean certain medical equipment
- Start IV drips or give medication
- Monitor medication and a patient's response
- Prepare and give injections and enemas
- Supervise nursing assistants and aides, and other LPNs

To become a licensed practical nurse, you don't need an associate's or bachelor's degree to practice, although formal training will be required. Most state-approved LPN programs are approximately 1 to 2 years in length. According to the *Occupational Outlook Handbook,* most programs include both classroom study (covering basic nursing concepts such as anatomy, physiology, medical-surgical nursing, pediatrics, obstetrics nursing, pharmacology, nutrition, and first aid) and clinical practice in a hospital setting[1]. Upon completion of the program, the NCLEX-PN must be taken and passed in order to receive licensing.

According to the Bureau of Labor Statistics the following statistics is the expected pay rate in each respective industry for a licensed practical nurse:

Median Annual Wages for LPNs and LVNs in the Top Industries[5]	
Nursing and residential care facilities	$43,700
Home healthcare services	43,670
Government	43,480
Hospitals; state, local, and private	41,400
Offices of physicians	38,150

To obtain further information and statistics on becoming a licensed practical nurse, please visit the following link: Bureau of Labor Statistics for Licensed Practical Nurses.

http://1.usa.gov/1TXaqJu

Registered Nurses Job Description

Registered nurses are nurses that have completed and graduated from a state (&country)-approved, nursing program and have successfully completed and passed the NCLEX-RN test and obtained licensing[2].

The job of a registered nurse involves the following:

- Record patients' medical histories and symptoms
- Administer patients' medicines and treatments
- Set up plans for patients' care or contribute to existing plans
- Observe patients and record the observations
- Consult and collaborate with doctors and other healthcare professionals
- Operate and monitor medical equipment

- Help perform diagnostic tests and analyze the results
- Teach patients and their families how to manage illnesses or injuries
- Explain what to do at home after treatment
- Work as part of a healthcare team with physicians and other healthcare specialists
- Supervise licensed practical nurses, nursing assistants and home health aides

To become a registered nurse there are one of three educational paths: a Bachelor of Science in nursing (B.S.N.), an associate's degree in nursing (A.D.N.) or a diploma from an approved nursing program.

The Bachelor of Science in nursing (B.S.N.) program usually takes about 4 years to complete. This program consist of the basic nursing courses (anatomy, physiology, microbiology, chemistry, nutrition, psychology, social and behavioral sciences, as well as liberal arts) and additional education in the physical and social sciences, communication, leadership and critical thinking and offers more clinical experience in nonhospital settings[3].

The associate's degree of nursing usually takes about 2 to 3 years to complete. This program consist of the basic nursing courses (anatomy, physiology, microbiology, chemistry, nutrition, psychology, social and behavioral sciences, as well as liberal arts) and a few other academic courses.

Upon completion of any of the previous programs mentioned, the NCLEX-RN must be taken and passed in order to receive licensing.

According to the Bureau of Labor Statistics the following statistics is the expected pay rate in each respective industry for a registered nurse:

Median Annual Wages for RNs in the Top Industries[4]	
Government	$70,540
Hospitals; state, local, and private	68,490
Home healthcare services	63,810
Nursing and residential care facilities	59,840
Offices of physicians	59,550

To obtain further information and statistics on becoming a registered nurse, please visit the following link: Bureau of Labor Statistics for Registered Nurses.

http://1.usa.gov/1TzKedl

Advice on Choosing Between a LPN and RN Program

I'll leave you with two words of advice on choosing a career path of becoming a nurse.

The first thing is to find a reputable state(&country)-approved program, that offers a LPN program, 2-year RN (A.D.N.) program, LPN to RN bridge program, and a B.S.N. program at the least and that have a high rate of students passing the NCLEX exams. This way if you choose to start with a LPN program, you will always have the opportunity for further advancement by enrolling in more advanced programs.

Secondly, if you start with and complete the LPN program and pass the NCLEX-PN, you can start to work immediately. And if you decide to go back to school to complete a more advanced program, your job may have a tuition reimbursement program that will help you to pay for your schooling, while at the same time you are gaining valuable experience.

Chapter 9. Conclusion

I hope that you've found this book to be thoughtful, informative and helpful, in making your decision to become a certified nursing assistant. Personally, I've thoroughly enjoyed the medical field and being a certified nursing assistant. It has its ups and downs, but at the end of the day, it's good to know that you've improved the quality of someone's life for the better and hopefully, one day someone will do the same for you.

Thank you for the purchase of this book and may you go far in your career.

Please visit our website and sign-up to be a member:
http://www.cnanationwide.com

Chapter 10. Bibliography or Citations

(Chapter 1-1) **http://bit.ly/1XBWqdz**
http://www.dementiatoday.com/experience-12-minutes-alzheimers-dementia/

(Chapter 3-1)
https://www.osha.gov/SLTC/medicalfirstaid/recognition.html

(Chapter 3-2) **http://bit.ly/1XW7gvr**
http://cpr.heart.org/AHAECC/CPRAndECC/AboutCPRFirstAid/UCM_473210_About-CPR-FirstAid.jsp

(Chapter 3-3)
http://cpr.heart.org/AHAECC/CPRAndECC/Training/HealthcareProfessional/BasicLifeSupportBLS/UCM_476233_BLS-for-Healthcare-Providers---Classroom.jsp

(Chapter 3-4) **http://bit.ly/1U0bixb**
http://work.chron.com/difference-between-patient-care-technician-cna-18240.html

(Chapter 4-1) https://en.wikipedia.org/wiki/Nursing_home_care

(Chapter 4-2)
http://beta.merriam-webster.com/dictionary/nursing%20home

(Chapter 4-3) https://en.wikipedia.org/wiki/Nursing_agency

(Chapter 4-4)
http://www.carepathways.com/HC-types-of-agencies.cfm

(Chapter 5-1)
http://www.aoa.acl.gov/Aging_Statistics/index.aspx

(Chapter 5-2)
http://www.bls.gov/ooh/healthcare/nursing-assistants.htm

(Chapter 5-3)
http://www.bls.gov/ooh/healthcare/nursing-assistants.htm#tab-6

(Chapter 5-4)
http://longtermcare.gov/costs-how-to-pay/costs-of-care/

(Chapter 5-5) http://www.payscale.com/

(Chapter 5-6)
http://www.bls.gov/oes/current/oes311014.htm#st

(Chapter 5-7)
http://www.bls.gov/oes/current/oes311014.htm#st

(Chapter 5-8) **http://bit.ly/1qap41l**
http://www.payscale.com/research/US/Job=Certified_Nurse_A
ssistant_(CNA)/Hourly_R ate

(Chapter 8-1)
https://en.wikipedia.org/wiki/Licensed_practical_nurse

(Chapter 8-2) https://en.wikipedia.org/wiki/Registered_nurse

(Chapter 8-3)
http://www.bls.gov/ooh/healthcare/registered-nurses.htm#tab-4

(Chapter 8-4)
http://www.bls.gov/ooh/healthcare/registered-nurses.htm#tab-5

(Chapter 8-5) **http://1.usa.gov/1TXaqJu**
http://www.bls.gov/ooh/healthcare/licensed-practical-and-
licensed-vocational-nurses.htm#tab-5

www.ingramcontent.com/pod-product-compliance
Lightning Source LLC
Chambersburg PA
CBHW070227210526
45169CB00023B/1004